Stay Fit for Life:

Everything You Need to Get a Slim, Fit and Healthy Body

Patricia Williams

Copyright

Contents

Introduction

Wouldn't it be wonderful if life allowed you to eat whatever you want without gaining a single pound? It would be bliss wouldn't it?

You no longer have to worry about watching your weight, or searching through the refrigerator for a low-calorie snack because you're almost at your limit, or having to exercise those excessive calories off, or having to painfully decide whether or not you should eat that delicious cake sitting on your kitchen table waiting for you to come take a piece of it.

Unfortunately, life does not work that wonderfully because even if you didn't have to worry about the calories that you're gaining, then you would have to worry about the type of food that you're putting in your body.

Well, it's obvious by now that losing weight isn't easy. If this is your first diet then welcome aboard and hope that you'll stay on.

If this isn't your first diet then please continue and figure out the reason as to why your previous methods have not worked. Yes it does suck that losing weight isn't as easy as gaining weight.

It's harder to put off the amount of calories that you're eating per day than to gain additional calories in one day. We all want weight loss to be simple and it has been wrongly emphasized that weight loss works best when you eat less and work out more.

It's also been wrongly emphasized that diet pills will help you lose weight. Honestly, if the concept of weight loss was that simple then how would obesity be possible?

Sadly, obesity is possible and it's occurring on a daily basis. The reason is due to the high level of fast food restaurants located all around us. However, before we can move into the deeper portion of the weight loss system, we have to know the basis of why our bodies make it difficult for us to lose weight in the first place.

The reason is simply due to our ancestors. That's right. It's their fault and the environment they were raised in. Due to the lack of available food back then, our ancestors made sure to eat as much food as possible before their starvation period started again.

From there, their body starts to store what was known as fat. In order for them to survive, their bodies were never programmed to set a limit on the amount of fat they could accumulate all at one time.

Unfortunately, now in the present day era, we no longer suffer through the starvation period. We have plenty of foods available to us and it's both cheap and easy to obtain.

Therefore, if we try to move our body into the starvation period in order to lose weight, we'll actually be gaining more weight because our metabolism will slow down and our remaining muscle will turn into fat in order for our body to save us from dying.

Even if we were to exercise on a consistent basis in order to rid ourselves of the excessive fat, we will still have to maintain an extreme level of willpower in order to continue on the diet trend. Of course, what can rapid weight loss also do to our immune system?

A few risks that you should definitely keep in mind are: kidney failure, depression, anorexia, and anxiety. A bigger risk that you should also keep in mind is that once you've lost all that weight in that short amount of time, it can bounce right back at you times two.

So before you move those fingers of yours to flip the page, ask yourself this: do you want to move quickly with difficultly, or do you want to move slowly and easily? Think about it for a moment because you wouldn't want to start emphasizing the "die" in the word diet.

Chapter 1: Weight Loss Negativity

This is the first chapter; the chapter where you will start to gain the basic knowledge of why you have failed before and what you shouldn't do so that you don't fail again.

Since you're here, it means that you have accepted the fact that weight loss will take time. You will not be able to lose weight quickly but slowly, and what you are doing is making a life long contract to lose weight.

That's right, this program is life long. It means that the moment you start on this program, you can never back out ever again. Of course, life long doesn't sound that bad.

After a few months, this program will become your secondary habit. It's going to change you and it's going to help you. You're going to feel healthier and your body is going to become fit, slim, and firm. Once you start seeing results, you won't even want to go back to your past self.

So this chapter is going to focus entirely on what you can't do and what you shouldn't do during your weight loss period. Discard any previous diet plans that you have had before away into the trash and from your mind.

The fact that it hasn't been working gives you a sign that it shouldn't be bothered with. All those pills and expensive food subscriptions that tell you how you can lose weight are all wrong.

This is your body that you want to change. Any program that will allow you to lose weight at a quick rate will not work for a long time because change requires time. Therefore, this program will be based mainly on time and food.

What we will be going over in this chapter are the rules of the diet game. This will be an important section because rules are necessary for success. That's probably why you didn't succeed with your previously diet plan, because it didn't have proper rules that you had to abide to.

However, before that, we will be taking a look at the type of people that you see everywhere in the streets. If you think that other skinny people are unfair, then you are in for a real treat as to why they are what they are.

Finally, we will end the chapter with the myth game. Myths are always fun to read simply because it clears up any form of misunderstandings that you've had before or any additional questions that you've never had answered. So, with these topics ready to go, let's start.

Types of Skinnies

Any overweight person would be jealous of any underweight person. However, any underweight person would be jealous of any overweight person. It's kind of funny how that process works doesn't it? The issue with those who are overweight is that they are trying hard to lose weight.

Whereas, the issue with those who are underweight is that they are trying to gain weight. Now you're probably wondering, "If they're already skinny, why do they want to be fatter?" The answer is simple, "Because it might be a health problem."

If we were to take a look at how unfair life can be, we should also take a look at the different types of skinny people in the world. Unfortunately, being thin also has its categories.

What you need to keep in mind is that not everyone is skinny and thin because they want to be. Sometimes, it's out of their will and, in their world, it's unfair to them too.

Remember, at the end of the day, you are not fat because you're being punished. You are fat because you are eating too much, working out too less, and not properly watching your weight. After all, "you are what you eat".

The Hard Workers

These are the type of people who are going through the exact same problem that you are. They don't want to stay overweight and therefore, they have to work to maintain their current weight. They keep a tab on everything that they eat and they maintain a healthy and active lifestyle.

They keep their health at the top of their priority list and always stay alert as to what type of food they're about to eat. If you think that it's going to be hard for you to keep it going for a few months? These people have been going through the same diet for years. Yet, no worries, they're used to it by now and, soon, you will too.

The Lucky Bunch

These are the type of people that you really want to be. They're the really lucky ones and the ones that you should feel jealous against. These are the type of people who barely have to work in order to maintain their weight.

In a sense, they're the naturally thin type of people. They only eat when they're hungry and they won't have to eat a lot in order to be full. It's the perfect type of balance for them because they won't under-eat and over-eat.

They'll eat the right portions at the right time and if they want to eat junk food, it'll only take a little bit of exercise to lose those excessive calories.

The Ones Who Want to be You

These are the type of people who wants to gain the amount of weight that you have. Well, they want to gain weight. They just don't want to be overweight. If you have been jealous at these types of people who can eat whatever they want at any time then think again.

The only reason why they can eat anything they want is because their body digests their food too quickly. These are the type of people who were born with fast metabolism.

Although that might seem like a blessing to have, it's a danger source for these people. The simple reason is because they are underweight and are prone to harmful symptoms like anorexia, or acid flux.

The Diet Rules

Technically, you don't really need rules when you move yourself into a diet. However, rules are essential for any type of success.

Rules make it easier on your part to know what not to do and what to do for any work. That is why dieting has rules established for you. Without them, you will have to go through many other trial and errors that you don't want to face.

Make sure that you pay close attention to what the rules are. Like all rules, one mistake can cause you a lot of damage. You might even hit a plateau on the way if you were to break one rule.

So be careful and be conscious of what you're doing. After a while, these rules will be etched into your mind and you'll be following them without realizing.

Have a Plan

When you start your diet plan without a plan, you are starting a disaster. Dieting is not a process that you can just "wing" like a school assignment and expect to pass.

Dieting takes planning, dedication, and calculation. If math was your most hated subject back in school, then sorry to say that it's going to become your greatest friend the moment you start dieting.

Every single day that you are dieting, you have to take note of your calorie intake. You have to plan out what you're going to eat, when are you going to eat it, the portion size, and how many times you're going to eat per day. It's always good to eat 5 times a day, 3 main meals and 2 snack-time meals.

You're also going to have to plan out how to train yourself to resist food that you want to eat when you can't eat them. This isn't about endurance as much as it is about wit.

When you are sad, depressed, or feeling bored, you tend to flock to the fridge and eat. Well, careful planning would have prepared you to empty out your house from any type of junk food available.

Think about it, the amount of times you step out of your comfort zone and into the fridge is about 5 times a day. If you eat junk food about that many times a day, you're never going to lose the first 5 pounds of your diet.

Make sure you can carefully and precisely. Don't forget to create a backup plan. It'll be especially useful for when you move yourself out into the real world and into the supermarket with a vast amount of diabetes and obesity upon every self.

Be Positive

When you start your first 2 weeks of the diet plan, you're going to feel excited and persistent. You're going to want to do everything right and you're going to want to follow all the rules that you should do.

It's going to be the most motivated 2 weeks of your life until you hit the rest of the month. By then, you're going to start feeling tired and unmotivated.

Sometimes, you might just want to bust out a bag of chips and eat away your hunger because you're too lazy to prepare a new meal for yourself. The problem is, is that you can't because, if you do, then you have repacked what you tried to lose.

You have to remember to stay positive throughout the whole program. Negativity can cause you to crave a lot of unhealthy foods and it's going to ruin your plan of success.

Make sure that you're going into this program fully knowing that you will indeed hit a wall almost every step of the way. It's not going to be smooth sailing once you've got the boat going. You're going to hit storms along the way.

As mentioned, don't think that winging it is going to help you. It might work out in the first few weeks, but it's not going to work out forever.

If you know perfectly well what you're getting yourself into then the whole plan will feel 10x easier than it would be.

Don't be like others who tend to plunge into a program without expecting any setbacks. Be mentally and physically prepared for the worse case scenario. Don't whine and complain either because it's not going to get you anywhere.

Be Conscious of Your Actions

Don't try fooling yourself about what you're eating. If that bag of chips is labeled 200 calories then it is 200 calories. Don't brush that 200 off of your calorie records by saying that 200 is nothing.

In weight loss, every calorie counts. Even 1 calorie can cause you to go over your daily intake limit. Women should be extra careful in this category. They tend to tell themselves that it's nothing and that everything will be fine.

Newsflash, it won't be. Women tend to be more conscious about their weight more than men do. So why is it that they tend to fool themselves about food more than men do? That's a question best left unanswered.

The point is, don't justify your actions with an excuse. If you want to eat because you're hungry then eat a fruit. Little things do matter even if you don't want them to. It sucks, but it's life.

Make Realistic Goals

Now, you were taught at a very young age that there is no such thing as a stupid idea. However, if someone hasn't broken it to you yet, then it's time for it to be broken now.

There is such thing as a stupid idea and the same applies to goals. Although goals can't be differentiated by intelligence, it can be differentiated between something that's possible to do and something that's impossible to do.

If you're making an impossible goal then you're not going to get anywhere. Something impossible would be like losing 10 pounds in a week.

If you're goal included the additional health factor then it's never going to happen. The safest way to lose weight is 1-2 pounds a week. Any more and you're being too brutal.

Realistic goals are possible goals. They are accomplishable and they are detailed. Realistic goals can be losing 2 pounds per week.

However, you're going to have to be way more specific than that. How are you going to lose 2 pounds per week? What are your plans for exercises? When are you going to exercise?

What type of exercises will you do for this day? What type of food do you have planned out for yourself?

In the beginning, planning every detail will be a pain to keep up with. However, after a while, it will take you less than 5 minutes to plan your weekly calendar. Of course, your schedule will not be 100% accurate.

There's always setbacks, and off happenings that you won't expect and that's OK. The purpose of a schedule is to keep you on track for a regular day.

Keep Going

Just because you dedicate yourself into losing weight, doesn't mean that losing weight has to be on your mind every single day.

If you think that weight loss is an all or nothing game that requires your full concentration then you're wrong. You do not have to be perfect at managing your weight into order to lose weight.

It's expected that you will hit plateaus regardless of what you do. If you came up with the idea that one mistake will ruin your whole plan then scratch it.

Many people tend to make the mistake of thinking that it's ok for you to do whatever you want for the rest of the day because you've already messed up. No, that is not how dieting works.

Remember, in a diet, every calorie counts. Why are you adding more calories into your body just because you happen to accidentally add a few now?

If you ate a piece of cake that was unplanned, doesn't mean that you should allow yourself to eat another serving of ice cream. The proper idea is to immediately move back into your planned diet after eating that piece of cake.

The Myth Game

Myths are always fun to read up on for just about anything. Myths are basically false facts that many people have come to believe that it's true. You've probably heard a few of these myths during the course of your life, especially if you've been through the whole dieting process before.

Myths generally do not help you and may be the reason why your weight loss plans have failed in the past. Most of these myths are created because people want to quickly lose their weight.

Therefore, some of these myths can be harmful to you and your body. In addition, these myths will only help you lose weight momentarily. They will not help you in the long run and you will surely regain what you've lost.

So if you've been following one of the myths listed here in the past, you now know why you couldn't lose weight before.

Note that only a few myths are listed here and that there are probably more out there. This is only the generally list that most people have probably heard before.

Genetics

Normally, genetics do play an important role in shaping your body, and personality, and everything else that came with the baby package. However, one of the few aspects that genetics do not play a part of is the size of your body.

If you're fat then genetics has nothing to do with that. You cannot blame your genes for making you fat. You can only blame your eating habits.

However, you can blame your genes for giving you a slow metabolism. Nevertheless, you should always be conscious of the food that you're eating.

The size of your stomach is based on the amount of food that you're eating minus the amount of time you spend exercising. If your exercise time is equal to zero then it's no wonder you're prone to gaining weight. This, in turn, brings us to our next myth.

Slow Metabolism

Most people are born with either an average metabolism or a slow metabolism. It's actually quite rare that people will be born with a fast metabolism. However, your metabolism shouldn't become the factor that stops you from losing weight.

Your metabolism is the level of speed your body takes to produce energy. When young, everyone will have a different metabolism rate. However, during old age, everyone will have a slow metabolism.

Of course, that doesn't mean that you can't change up the speed of your metabolism. In fact, metabolism rate is not fixed and can change depending on how much you exercise and the type of food that you eat. The more active you are and the healthier the food you eat, the faster your metabolism will be.

Skipping on Meals

If you believe in the notion that starvation equals success then you are dead wrong. For one reason, starving yourself only makes you fatter. When you stop eating despite being hungry, your body will go into its defense mode and start converting your muscles into additional fat.

So the whole purpose of starving yourself in order to lose fat has backfired. In addition to extreme hunger, your body will start craving foods that you shouldn't even be touching.

You're metabolism will slow down in order to preserve your energy and it's going to require a tremendous amount of willpower in order to stop yourself from taking a bite of the food in front of you. Note that skipping meals can also make you prone to other diseases and symptoms that you want to avoid.

Walking is Pointless

Walking is everything. Although walking may not burn as much calories as the typical workouts, it does help in burning some extra calories. You cannot say that walking does not work because, technically, walking is still an exercise.

Believe it or not, you are able to burn 250 calories a day if you were to walk 10 thousand steps a day. Although that may sound a lot, those steps will fly by quickly.

So instead of taking the car for a 2-3 minutes drive to a destination two blocks away, start walking there. You'll also help reduce the amount of pollution in our economy while you're at it.

Exercise is Everything

It doesn't matter what kind of weight loss program you are on, or how well your diet plan is, every successful weight loss program starts in the kitchen. Remember, food before exercise.

Of course, you can burn off a lot of calories at the gym doing intense cardiovascular and weight lifting workouts, but what decides how hard you have to work starts in the kitchen.

The amount of calories you take in depends on what type of food you are taking. The amount of calories you have to burn off depends on the type of food that you are eating.

If you think about it, you can work hard exercising your body to its limit, but your food choices can bounce those calories right back up within seconds.

Chapter 2: Weight Loss Positives

So now we'll be moving into the positive aspects of weight loss and what you can do to stay motivated with the program. Even though losing weight may seem like a difficult commitment to keep, it's actually quite easy to do.

If you have prepared your mind to conquer the most devastating set backs in your conquest to lose weight, you will have a much easier time conquering any major issues that you will face.

The best method of maximizing your chances of success is trial and error. This doesn't mean that you should approach weight loss with a mind full of mistakes planned out.

It means that if you mess up, learn from your mistakes. Take it as a lesson and don't feel bummed out about it. Mistakes produce growth and growth produces achievement.

So before you move on from your mistakes, always take a moment to figure out what you did wrong and what you will improve on next time.

In this chapter, we will go over making goals for a positive weight loss experience. Goals are essential for any type of success, and will help make your experiences much easier and less intimidating.

Then, we will take a look at how to stay motivated with the weight loss program. Finally, we will end the chapter by discussing what you can do to maintain good habits throughout the weight loss program.

Making Goals

Goals are always easy to make but hard to follow through. Many individuals tend to make 1-2 goals on a daily basis. However, only a handful of them will actually follow through with their goals.

The reason why is because they're either too unmotivated to follow through with their words or they're goals weren't specific enough for them to start.

A goal always needs to be specific, detailed, and realistic. Now nothing is impossible in life if you set your mind to it. However, there are things that you can't do within a short amount of time.

Losing weight is a goal, but it's not a detailed goal. Losing 2 pounds per week is a realistic goal, but its still missing extra details as to how are you going to lose those 2 pounds.

Losing more than 5 pounds per week is an unrealistic goal because it's too much work and it's going to cause damage to your body.

How do you know if your goal is a realistic goal? One question that you can ask yourself is, "Is it easy for me to do?" If you feel that the goal you've made is easy then it's a realistic goal. An unrealistic goal is one that seems too difficult to do and one that you won't feel motivated to accomplish.

The best part about goals is the fact that you don't have to focus on one main goal. You can set a main goal and branch it into small goals. Usually, main goals are long lasting goals that can take years to accomplish.

However, small goals will take either a day or a few weeks to complete. Not only that, but as you're working on your smaller goals, you are getting slower to your main goal.

Now, what we're going to talk about in this section is the characteristics of how to set an effective goal for the future. These are tips that will teach you the basis of making goals, and it will help make weight loss seem a lot easier than before.

Be Specific

This was already mentioned before so we will only move a little deeper into the concept. When you make a goal, you're basically making a statement of commitment.

It doesn't have to be like a contract where you have to sign your life away. Although, there might be those who would go that far just to make sure that they stick to their words.

Sometimes, everybody just needs a little push to start his or her goals since the first step is always the most difficult. The best method to starting a goal is to simply do it, and the best way to motivate yourself into doing it is to know what you're about to do.

During the goal making process, you have to take every factor into consideration. You have to mention when you will do the task, how long will it take you, where are you going to do it, and what time will you start.

Since we're on the weight loss subject, let's say that your goal was to lose 2 pound in one week. To answer the question of "when", you can mention a date or two - say Monday and Wednesday.

To answer the question of "how long", you can say for half an hour to an hour. "Where" can be at the gym and "what time" can be at 2 P.M.

So, when you put those pieces together, your goal will be something like this: Since my goal will be to lose 2 pounds this week, I will go to the gym at 2 P.M. on Monday and Wednesday for an hour. This is an example of a realistic and specific goal.

What makes that goal even better will be flexibility. Every great goal is flexible.

Since you cannot accurately determine what will happen the next day, you have to make sure that you are able to switch your schedule around in order to accomplish your goal.

So let's say that there was traffic on your way to the gym after you got off work and you're behind schedule by 10 minutes.

That's perfectly fine also because you can either cut down your gym time but still have the workout that you planned, or you can kick off the next item on the list for extra time at the gym. Of course, if you're going to skip another item on your schedule, make sure that it's not an important appointment.

Make Sure it's Doable

Is your goal doable? We talked about this earlier on about making realistic goals that you can easily accomplish. If your goal is easy and doable then you are on the right track to creating a successful goal.

Remember, you want to make a doable goal that won't kill you, or cause any harm to your body. The point of losing weight is to be healthy and to stay healthy.

Weight loss isn't a race. It's designed to improve your health, not to worsen it. Always start with easy goals before moving into harder goals. That way, you will get the hang of sticking to your word before you start making any difficult commitments.

Always imagine yourself succeeding before you start on your goals. For one thing, it's a motivational booster for when you actually start because you'll already feel a sense of accomplishment.

For a second reason, if you can imagine yourself succeeding then you know that it's a doable goal. Be honest with your imagination.

Make Progress

Are you sure that your goal can be tracked for progress. A good goal allows improvement. A bad goal gives you nothing.

When making a goal, you have to make sure that the end results will benefit you. If not then think of another one. You have to make sure that your goal leaves room for feedback and improvement.

Remember, a goal equals growth. If a goal does not match up to your needs then adjust it as much as you want until you feel satisfied. It is your progress and not anyone else's.

Stay Motivated

Motivation can be difficult to conjure for the most part. Normally, people find motivation to be easy to obtain when they first start out a new goal.

However, after pursuing that goal for about a month, majority of them start to die out. Then there are some who give up completely. It's often rare to see someone follow through with his or her plans until the end.

Anyhow, as mentioned before, once you pursue your diet program you are going to be making a life long goal. This is not temporary.

This is going to be for the rest of your life. Now that may sound intimidating for you right now and it may cause your motivation to die out a little.

However, you have to think about the choices given to you right here: would you rather stay unhealthy and fat, or would you rather stay slim, fit, and healthy for the rest of your life. Obviously, the second choice would be the best choice.

Unlike other diet plans that you've faced, this plan doesn't send you back into the drawing board once you're done. It makes you keep going and it keeps you feeling great.

You're no longer going to keep starting at base 1 once you've reached home run. You're going to keep running and never grow tired.

Of course, this program doesn't expect your 100% commitment. In fact, we would rather you not commit 100%. The reason why is because weight loss is not perfect. People are not perfect.

You're going to crave eventually and that's perfectly fine as long as you don't go overboard with the craving.

All you need to do is give at least 50% percent of your effort and 90% max. You may balance out the remaining percentage to do whatever you want with your food choices and your exercise routine.

As long as you feel that losing weight is easy and that you're motivated to continue, you are on the right track.

Also, you may even reward yourself for accomplishing your weight loss goals just as long as your reward doesn't include food.

Remember, even if you're on the diet plan, it doesn't mean that you should revolve your life around food. You are free to eat whatever, whenever you want as long as you are conscious of what you're doing.

So why spend your reward on food when you can spend it buying a new pair of shoes at the mall, or a new laptop, or even a vacation. As long as you are keeping up with your diet plan, you are free to do whatever you please.

Your Habits

Habits can either make or break you. The common saying of "old habits die hard" isn't emphasized because people think it's a nice saying.

It's emphasized because it's true. Since old habits die hard, they can also die with you. Having bad habits can damage you, but having good habits will make your life easier.

If you have any bad habits that you want to get rid of then now's the time to start if you haven't done so.

It can be tricky to get rid of an old habit but it's doable. Usually, old habits die out when new habits come in. So the solution is to make a new habit.

Although that may seem difficult to do, know that any repeated pattern of action will become a habit overtime. So if you're sticking to a proper schedule of repeated patterns then one of your to-dos will become a new habit for you before you know it.

Which brings us to the next topic: making a daily to-do list. You're going to need this if you want to continue staying healthy and consistently with your diet.

Making schedules might've given you a headache before but an agenda will become your best friend starting now. Buy a small agenda if you don't have one yet.

It's always good to buy the type that you can write in, and it's ever better if the time is spread out for you. Spend time planning out your schedule for the next day every night. After a while, that's going to become a habit. You'll realize that having a schedule will help make your life easier than before.

Chapter 3: Failing and Succeeding

Now we all have our moments of failure and success. You can't have one without the other. In order to succeed we have to first fail. That is how we grow as human beings in wisdom and in experience.

That's why, in this short chapter, we will discuss the stages of failing and succeeding the diet game. You're going to have to expect failure before you start making progress.

Everything will seem difficult at first, but as long as you keep going then your success will pay off. Afterwards, we will make a quick discussion about why we are so addicted to certain foods and what the real world has in store for us before we close off the chapter.

Hitting the Dead End

After your first few months of the weight loss program, you are going to experience what is known as a plateau.

A plateau is basically a dead end. It's when you've reached the wall of your goal and you have to figure out a way to conquer that wall in order to keep going.

Like all walls, there are small walls that you can hop over and there are big walls that you're going to have to break through.

The smaller walls aren't going to be an issue in your journey to losing weight. However, the big walls will. In this section, we will be taking a look at the two types of walls that you will encounter and what you can do to deal with them.

The Mini-Plateaus

The mini-plateaus are the smaller walls that you don't have to worry about much during your dieting process. These plateaus come and go and will do very little harm to your progress so far.

You do not have to worry about them much because they will normally away within 2-3 days. The reason why they aren't important is because you're probably experiencing the lazy days, or the days where you don't feel like you want to do anything.

Normally, when those days occur, they will only last for 1-2 days. However, there's always an after effect from those feelings, which will probably add another extra day to your plateau.

Of course, that doesn't mean that you should let it go and wait for it to subside. If you let it sink then it can turn into a lengthy-plateau, and you do not want to deal with those. The best method to getting rid of these mini walls is to simply continue on with your life.

Since it's only a minor issue, it's best to simply ignore it and continue your diet like you've always been. Eventually, you'll be back up on your feet as if nothing had happen.

The Big Plateaus

These are the plateaus that are going to cause you some effort to get rid of. They are the big walls and will usually last for more than three weeks.

These walls are a lot more difficult to ignore compared to the smaller walls, as it will not be easily broken. Note that once you've hit these walls, it's time to take action.

There are four main steps that you can take in order to get rid of the big plateaus. It's not as if you will face all of these but it's more of a list where you can pick and choose your issues and solutions.

Excessive Calories

Are you making sure that you're recording the proper amount of calories that you are supposed to consume per day?

Remember that every calorie counts and if you try to sneak in even a basic 100, your body will automatically know. The point of losing weight is so that you would watch your weight.

The fact that you're trying to sneak in extra calories as if it isn't a big deal isn't doing much for your benefit.

If you want to add in extra calories here and there then that's perfectly fine and up to your decision. However, you should at least record the amount that you're eating so that you can have the accurate amount of calories that you're taking in every day.

This way, you at least know what you can work off so your body doesn't start preserving those extra calories as fat.

If you don't know the right amount of calories that you're eating, you can always guesstimate. Although guesstimating is fine, it'll only work if you're making progress with your weight loss.

Be realistic with the calories in each food when you're guesstimating. If anything, you can always guess more calories than what it could've been to be sure that you don't pass your calorie limit.

Exercise Routines

How are you exercising? Are you doing it consistently? What about the routines? Are those consistent? The sometimes annoying part about our body is the fact that it can grow accustom to the same routine all the time.

If you tend to perform the same exercise routine on a consistent basis then your body will grow accustom to the workout and it will be harder for you to burn calories. The best method for fixing this issue is to add a variety to your exercise routine.

Let's say your normal exercise routine is to jog two miles a day, three days a week. So, what you should do to make sure that you're burning the right amount of calories that you want to is to change up that routine.

You can start either jogging three or four miles a day for three times a week, or for three to four miles for four times a week. The choice is up to you. Try to switch up your routines every five weeks for the best results.

Also, don't only focus on one type of workout. If you haven't done weights already, start them. It's a good break from cardiovascular workouts and it'll help make your body fit and firm.

You're not only going to burn off extra calories, you're also going to be shaping your body into the form you want.

Re-establish You Calorie Limit

Maybe the reason why you can't seem to lose any more weight from where you are now is because you need to change up your amount of calorie intake.

It means that your body is getting smaller and, therefore, your calorie intake will also become smaller. Normally, this would only happen after you've lost your first 20 pounds or so. This is a good sign and will require only a slight change in your diet to fix the issue.

You have two options: to exercise more or to eat fewer calories.

Take a Complete Break

Sometimes, when you are working yourself too hard, your body needs a break. The same goes with weight loss. If you've been losing a lot of weight on a consistent basis, and there are no issues with your diet and workouts then it's about time you stop and relax.

Start eating whatever you want again, but watch what you eat at the same time. You only want to take about a week vacation from dieting because any longer might cause you to crave that freedom.

Plus, a week is good enough if you are going to allow yourself to eat whatever you want. You are going to gain weight again from this method but that is why you shouldn't let it drag longer than a week.

It's enough time for your body to reset its metabolism and for you to relax from your hard work.

Why We Are Addicted

Did you ever wonder why we are so addicted to unhealthy foods while we can easily disregard the healthy ones? We obviously know what kind of food we're eating and what it can do to our body in the long run.

However, that is the least of our worries because all we want is that momentary goodness.

Well, the reason why unhealthy food is so addicting is because those foods are loaded with sugar, fat, and salt. Those are the three main ingredients for making you want more of what's unhealthy for you.

Not to mention the added chemicals that we can barely pronounce. The point is, these types of foods are designed to make you want to crave more.

Haven't you noticed how when you reach into those potato chip bags for some, you end up reaching into them again for more. It means that those ingredients are working, but your health is not benefitting.

Companies know what you want to eat and they're willing to make you crave it as long as they're the ones making the profit.

They are willing to advertise their food anywhere as long as you will buy it. Don't forget, whenever you buy any type of junk food, it's your loss and the company's victory.

The Real World

The real world is with too much temptation hidden around every shelf and every kitchen, and if you were to try to resist those temptations then you will only be making a fool of yourself.

We all want to be able to bask in the glory of eating junk food to our hearts content simply because junk foods taste better than healthy foods.

Of course, the only reason why it's called junk food is because it only fills our body with junk. So what can we do in order to rid ourselves of our temptations for unhealthy foods? We prepare ourselves.

When you go out into the real world, you need to prepare yourself for the vast amount of junk food available to you.

Those foods are easy to get and those foods are harmful. You need to come up with strategies that will help you combat these types of food everywhere you go, especially if you're planning any type of road trips.

Road trips are usually the number one reason for weight gain. Since you're constantly on the road without much civilization, you need food that can last for a long time.

Usually, the situation would call for junk food. However, there are healthy foods out there that can last for a long time on the road. That's when you have to figure out which ones.

You always want to pack healthy foods with you for any trip and it's always good to make a list before you head off to the store to buy them too.

By making a grocery list, you will only be shopping for food that you need without wasting time wandering around the aisle to find food.

If you're ever eating at a restaurant then consider taking leftovers home. Being at a restaurant doesn't mean that you have to finish everything on your plate.

Always take note of where you're going and what types of food will be available around you. If you're at a new location and you haven't done your research then it's time to make use of the free Internet around you.

Remember that you should always try to avoid eating at an all-you-can-eat buffet. Those places are the home of weight gainers.

Additional tips that you should keep in mind when eating out in the real world is to plan the meal that you want to eat. If you know the name of the restaurant that you're going to eat at then it's best to do research on it before hand.

Find out what type of food they serve and how many calories are each plate, if possible. That way, you will have an idea as to how many calories you will consume.

Once arrive at the restaurant, try to see if they are flexible with food choices. If they are, then ask them to replace some calorie-dense items on their menu for additional vegetables.

If they don't allow you to do that then the best method is to only eat half of what is given to you. If they are willing to automatically to-go half of your plate before you receive it then it will be easy for you to finish your plate.

If you want to be extreme about it then there's always the option of throwing the other half of the food away. Of course, that would be a waste of money and food at the same time.

If push comes to shove, you can always spoil your appetite before your food arrives. You may eat something at home before you arrive to the restaurant, or you may drink a lot of water as you're waiting for your food.

Water is a good method to make yourself seem full when you are trying to eat less. Also, in order to ensure that you will be full, chew your food slowly.

When you eat too fast, your body won't be able to digest it as quickly. However, if you were to take your time and eat, you are giving your body enough time to digest a part of what you've eaten.

Chapter 4: Basic Healthy Workouts

It can become difficult for just about anyone to maintain their weight, especially when they have no clue on where to go.

Sadly, the failure rate presented in the USA for those who try to lose weight is 99.5%, which is basically almost everybody.

So what does the remaining .5% of people do in order to succeed? They remain active and exercise daily.

Although this chapter is dedicated to discussing about the different type of workouts that you can do to stay active, we are also going to be taking a look at how to successfully maintain your current weight as well as the maximum amount of calories you need per day.

Successful Maintenance

Commitment to any type of exercise may be difficult at first due to your scheduling and motivation. However, once you've made exercising a habit, it's going to be one part of your life that you won't want to skip out on.

Sure it may seem tiring and you might not be able to deal with the sweating and constant soreness. Nevertheless, you will feel great after every workout. Your body will be healthy, and you will feel healthy. It's an easy way to lose weight and you'll always feel active and on the move regardless of where you are.

In addition, there will be more flexibility in your diet. You can't always eat the same healthy food every single day. You're going to crave for sweets throughout your diet and that is why exercising is so useful.

Besides, when you feel active, your mind will clear up. You can think clearer and you'll be less stressed out than before.

Exercise also makes you stronger. Eventually those twenty-pound package of water that you had trouble lifting before will soon be nothing to you.

Ladies, you will start gaining muscles in place of your fat. However, if you're doing the proper exercise, you can choose where your muscles will show.

Of course, it's always better to have muscles rather than fat. Although muscles will increase your weight by a little, it's better to have a firm body rather than a flabby one.

Since exercising may seem difficult to start in the beginning, it's always good to have a few principals that can keep you going. These are going to be your daily motivators and it's going to help get you into shape.

Be Goal Oriented

When you plan your daily schedule, always try to plan time to exercise. You are not expected to work out every day, and it's recommended that you don't anyways.

The best workout plan is to exercise about 3 or 4 times a week for about half an hour to an hour each workout. If you've been sticking to your goals and accomplishing like you're supposed to then you are someone who is goal oriented.

Therefore, it's expected that you should start planning exercise routines into your schedule so you would be forced to do them. It will be your new goals and, once you've gotten used to exercising, it will become your new habits.

When planning, make sure you switch up between cardiovascular and weight lifting exercises. You are not expected to do both on the same day.

You may plan to jog for an hour one day and weight lift for an hour another day. As long as you are consistent with your workout then you will be fine. Remember to switch up your routine once every so often.

If you keep doing the same workout, your body will become adjusted to it and it will be harder for you to lose weight. Always remember to have a little note of what type of workout you will be doing on our active days.

That way, you can save time by already knowing what you will do rather than contemplating about it while you're there.

Balance it Out

Make sure that you are able to balance out the timing for your exercises and your food choices. Just because you exercise, doesn't mean that you can eat whatever you want.

Exercise only helps if you want to relax with your food choices once in a while, not all the time. Believe it or not, you don't burn as much weight in one hour to allow yourself to consume a large Frappuccino and a piece of cake within a few minutes.

You need to keep both balanced in order to maintain your weight.

Also, remember, this is a life long commitment. Once you've reached your obtained weight, you have to keep it the way it is and it's going to require the same amount of effort as before.

Don't ever stop half way and don't ever over pack your schedule. You will get tired after each workout and you will feel sore the day after.

Give yourself a light schedule whenever you're planning on doing intense workouts for the day. The reason why it's recommended that you exercise every other day is so your body can rest the next day.

Gain Supporters

One of the easiest ways to maintain motivation throughout the beginning of your exercise habits is to have a partner with you. Find a friend who supports your effort to lose weight and ask them if they are willing to exercise with you.

You want to find multiple friends and not just one because everyone else may have different schedules. Try to work your schedule around with theirs and ask them if they would do the same.

If you now someone who tends to stay consistent with their workouts, try to see if you can ask them about the type of exercises you should do and what is a good starting point for you. If they are exercise fanatics then they will be glad to help.

If you feel that none of your friends are wiling to help you out or that they're mocking you, it's about time you start finding new friends who can give you the motivational boost and support that you need.

Remember, friends are a choice. You can choose who you want to hang out with and you can choose who you want to leave.

Of course, leaving a friend that you've known for a few years may be harsh. However, what are you benefiting from them if they can't be there to support you in your time of need?

Necessary Calories

Before you head off to your workouts, you need to know the amount of calories that you should consume on a daily basis. This way, you can better plan your workouts to match with the foods that you're eating on a daily basis.

If you know that you're going to be eating more calories on a particular day, you also need to know what type of exercises you can do in order to rid yourself of those extra calories.

If you allow excessive calories to seep through your body then your body can store it as fat.

Normally, for an average man, you are able to consume up to 2,900 calories and 2,100 calories for an average woman. However, these numbers are only used as a starting point for your body since calorie consumption will vary with each person.

In order to accurately measure the amount of calories you can consume per day, you have to take your schedule into consideration.

How active are you on a daily basis? Do you exercise consistently? If you tend to move around a lot during the day then you should add an extra 100 calories to your diet.

If not then take away an extra 100 from the average. It's always good to start small when adding or subtracting calories. That way, you're not going to risk the chance of consuming too much or too little.

Make sure that you never bother yourself with any type of diet pills thinking that it can help you lose some extra calories.

Most likely, those pills will only make you gain weight by stimulating your cravings. Also, those pills will affect your mood and health. Lose weight the natural way because you can't cheat your body.

Simple Cardiovascular Exercises

You should always take cardiovascular exercises into consideration for losing weight. It's the best method for getting rid of excessive fat around your body.

Cardiovascular exercises also help improve your health, and strengthen your lungs. So if you suffer through asthma, doing some cardiovascular exercises can help you overcome it. Of course, it's always best to consult to your doctor first if you're unsure.

There are plenty of cardiovascular exercises for you to choose from. If you're the type of person who hates running, be glad that running isn't your only option.

Depending on the length of your workout, you can burn between 300-600 calories. Note that the more you weight, the more calories you'll burn all at once compare to someone you weights less.

That's because those who weight less is already limited to what they can burn because of the lack of fat in their body.

Most of these exercises will range from half an hour to one hour. For every half an hour that you do these exercises, you will be burning about 300 calories, give or take.

A few good workouts would be hiking, swimming, basketball, or tennis. All of these can be done with another partner or a group of people.

For basketball and tennis, the workout is included with few minor rests in between. If you're a bike person, you'll only be burning about 300 calories every hour that you're biking, minus the resting interval within each hour.

If you decide to walk, then you would have to walk about an hour and a half in order to burn 300 calories. If you're speed walking then you might be able to burn the same amount in about an hour.

Of course, walking can take place anywhere and anytime throughout your day. If you take about 10,000 steps per day, you're already burning 250 calories.

Chapter 5: Basic Abs Workout

These workouts are mainly focus on weight lifting and are designed to train your stomach into the shape that you want it to be.

Even if you've lost the weight that you wanted, you should still try to maintain a thin firm stomach rather than a thin flabby one. There are other exercises designed to help you maintain the rest of your body.

However, those would require weights while abdominal workouts do not. In this chapter, we will only go over the abdominal workouts.

The reason why is because these are easy workouts to do even at your home and not everyone will have access to weights and a gym facility.

Make sure that you don't do these types of workouts every day. You always want to give your body a day's worth of rest after every workout so every other day will be a good plan.

In the beginning of your workouts, you will become very sore because your body is not used to the intensity. However, later on, your body will adjust to it.

That doesn't mean that you won't feel sore at all. It just means that you are used to the feeling so it will not affect you as much as before.

If you are not feeling any type of soreness the day after your workout, it means that you need to increase the intensity of it in order to obtain the full effect.

It will be difficult for you to obtain the firm body that you want in the beginning. It's definitely going to take some time before you still start seeing results.

However, once it's there, maintaining it will be a lot simpler. Make sure that whenever you do these exercises, you do them in intervals. For example, if you wanted to do a total of 50 sit ups then you would do then in sets of 5 with 10 sit ups per set.

This way, you are not risking the possible strain on your body and you will have a short break within each set. Each break between sets should only last for about 10 seconds before starting.

You would only take about a minute break when you are moving into a new workout. Practice these abdominal workouts every other day for about ten minutes max in order to obtain the best results.

Leg Thrust

This exercise is a two-part exercise that requires you to lay flat on your back with your head and shoulders raised off on the floor.

Your hands should be placed on the mat and near your hips and your legs should be raised until it is perpendicular to the floor.

From there, slowly lower your legs half way down before moving them back into its original position. Once you're back into your original position, thrust your hips off the floor and into the air.

Use your arms as your support if you need it. Repeat and continue this workout by doing 2 sets of 10 on your first time.

Abdominal Bicycles

For this workout, you're going to pretend that you're riding a bike. The only difference is that you're body is on the floor and you're pedaling air.

So, to start, lie on your back with your head and shoulders slightly lifted off the ground, your fingers touching your head, and your hips and knees perpendicular to the ground.

From there, move the left side of your body off the floor and towards each other and resume your normal position to do the right side of your body. The motions will be similar to riding a bicycle. You just have to remember to keep your legs straight as you're moving your legs in and out.

Reverse Crunches

Start by lying on your back on the floor with your legs bent and your head and shoulders slightly lifted off the ground. From there, slowly move your lower body off the ground and move your knees towards your head.

Do not push off and release this position immediately. You have to use your strength for this workout to work.

Abdominal Crunches

Abdominal crunches are similar to bicycles only that you are not required to move your legs. When starting, start in the same position as you would for reverse crunches.

Keep your arms bent and your hands placed on the side of your head. Then, move one side of your arm towards the opposite side of your leg. Do this slowly and hold it for one second before releasing and moving to the other side.

Abdominal Scissors

For this workout, you start by lying on your back with both your arms straight over your head and your legs slightly bent straight up.

There, bring your shoulders off the ground and your arms forward while bringing your legs and hips off the ground until both your legs and arms crosses one another. Hold for about two seconds and then release and repeat.

Breakdancer

For this workout, you have to position yourself on your hands and feet. Then, bring your right leg under and over your body so that your knee is near your left elbow.

From there, start jumping while switching to your left knee. Keep switching back and forth at a fast pace. It'll be like trying to breakdance. The only difference is that you're only doing part of the turn. Keep this going for about 1-2 minutes on your first try.

Planking

For this exercise, you'll have to lie completely on your front body. You are free to position your hand however you like as long as it provides you with the proper support that you need when you lift your body up.

Once in position, lift your body up so that your elbow is supporting your weight. Tighten up your abdominal muscles and hold that position for about one minute. This is a good ending workout to do before you close up for the day.

Chapter 6: Food for Thought

Did you know that food could do a lot to your mood and your outward appearance? If you tend to eat healthy food, your mood will brighten up because your body is receiving all of its proper nutrients.

You will feel stressed less often and your tolerance level will be higher. If you have the tendency to eat junk food most of the time, your mood will worsen and you will feel sluggish for the majority of the day.

In addition, eating healthy food can also improve the general outlook of your skin. You will have less of a chance for breakouts and your skin will age slower.

There are quiet a lot more benefits with eating healthy than unhealthy. Best of all, by having naturally healthy looking skin, you will no longer have to spend so much money on those expensive facial products ever again.

Nutrition Rules

In the beginning, we talked about how weight loss had its own set of rules that you need to follow if you want the best results.

Now, we're going to talk about the set of rules that you need to follow in order to obtain the best result in your diet.

Of course, in order to not overwhelm you we will only list the basic and most important rules here. These will be the general rules that you have to follow closely. It's going to be a pain in the beginning but you'll naturally remember them as time passes on.

Though, the number one rule that you should keep in mind is the fact that you can never lie to yourself. Make sure that you're counting your calories properly.

Take careful count of the amount of calories you're consuming and jolt them down before you begin to eat. If you wait until you've finished your meal, you might even forget to record it down because you'll be occupied with what's after.

Remember, you don't have to be 100% accurate with your calorie consumption. Sometimes, you're going to have to guesstimate and that's fine as long as you're not lying to yourself about what you're eating at the end of the day.

Take careful note of these tips whenever you plan your meals. It's going to act as a good starting point in your diet program.

Perfection is not Necessary

Dieting does not require you to be perfect since every natural diet plan was made with the expectation that you will crave and break.

If you were required to be perfect in order to lose weight then it would be impossible for half the population in the USA to lose weight. One aspect that people cannot deny the most is their desires.

Even extreme willpower will not last a lifetime. If you keep telling your mind to deny what you want the most then you will eventual desire the need to rebel from your own words. That is why you are not expected to be perfect in order to succeed in dieting.

This plan is suppose to help you relax and take things naturally. This plan is supposed to fix your bad habits by replacing them with new habits.

In order to do that, you have to feel comfortable. If a diet plan is placing too many limitations on you then it is not a good plan that you should stick it. However, you should always balance out your strictness level within your diet.

Always put a higher percentage of effort and a lower percentage of freedom. You want to be free to eat whatever you want, but you don't want to be too free so that you end up not losing weight at all.

Stay Within Your Limit

Always stay under the limit of your calorie consumption. Even a calorie over can be a big deal. Remember, every calorie counts. If you were to go over the limit of your daily calorie consumption then your body would take those excessive calories and stores it as fat.

Always look for natural food whenever you're planning your meal. Avoid canned and processed food at all times. Do not trust what the labeling says. Just by looking at the ingredient, you can already tell that it's not safe for your body.

Even if it's fruits or vegetable, going fresh and natural is the way to go. So start paying attention to food labeling nowadays, especially the ingredients that they were made out of.

Any food that contains ingredients that you can't pronounce is not something that you want to eat constantly.

Eat Consistently

Always try to eat about every 4 hours. Truth be told, people who tend to eat consistently will have an easier time losing weight than people who tend to skip out on their meals, which defeats the sole purpose of losing weight.

You cannot expect to lose weight if you were to starve yourself. If you forfeit your meal in order to be thinner then your plan will only backfire.

You will start feeling tired and dizzy and your cravings will spike up, causing you to eat unhealthy food in order to take away the hunger.

Because of that, you will be gaining even more calories because your body has already converted your muscle into fat, including the calories from what you just ate.

You want to eat consistent meals everyday, preferably at the same time if possible. Eat about five times a day, or six is you must – though five seems more appropriate: 3 main meals and 2 small meals.

Eat Protein

No matter what you're eating, whether it's a snack or a main dish, you should always try to add a little protein into your food. The reason why protein is so important to your body is the fact that it protects you from losing muscles.

So if you've been working out consistently, you do not what your efforts to go to waste because you didn't eat enough protein for the day.

In addition, protein also helps make you feel fuller during meals so you won't run the risk of overeating all the time.

Although protein is good for your body, too much of it can harm your body at the same time. That is why you should figure out how to measure the amount of protein you need in to consume on a daily basis so you don't run the risk of eating too much or eating too little.

The amount of protein you should take in also depends on how active you are on a daily basis. It's rated similar to calorie consumption but not as much.

The amount of protein that you should try to aim for each day should be one gram of protein per pound of your target body weight. Always try to do a little research as to which type of food contains protein and which food is highly recommended.

Fats

Fats can be a little tricky to handle. Throughout your whole life, you've been told that fats are bad for you and you are to avoid them. However, have you ever though about good fats that can actually help you?

Basically, there are two different types of fats. There are the omega 3 fats and there are the omega 6 fats. The bad fats that you've been told to avoid your whole life is the omega 6 fats.

Omega 6 fats are basically fats from processed foods. They come mainly from grains and processed vegetable oils, or anything that is pre-made and laid out for you in any store.

These are the fats that can kill you if you consume too much. Omega 3 fats, on the other hand, are the good type of fats for you.

Omega 3 fats actually help you age more slowly than those who have omega 6 fats in their body. These fats have long-term benefits for you and can help boost up your immune system and protect you from heart disease. It's also the type of fat that's useful for helping you lose weight.

Fruits and Vegetables

You always want to mix your food in with some fruits and vegetables. For the main dishes, try to add a variety of different vegetables with your food.

Even if you might dislike vegetables, you cannot hate all of them. Besides, there are plenty of ways to cook them. You can fry or boil vegetables if you don't enjoy eating them raw.

For fruits, it would be great if you were able to eat them as a snack rather than a part of your entre. It's always good to have at least 2-3 pieces of fruit per day, which is perfect because you can eat 2 per day during your snack time.

Of course, be wary of dry fruits. It's not recommended that you eat dry fruits compared to natural fruits. The reason is because dried fruits contain more calories than the natural kind. So, in turn, you will actually gain weight eating dried fruits.

Liquid

There are only two types of liquid beverages that you should allow yourself to drink every single day, and that is water and green tea.

Water has zero calories and will not fill your stomach up, but rather give you a momentary feeling of fullness. It's an especially useful trick to do when you want to eat less while dining out.

Tea is also good for your health and it's preferred that you drink green tea to any other types of tea.

You want to avoid any other beverages to the best of your abilities. If possible, don't drink sodas at all. If you're craving for it then once a few weeks is fine, but just not daily.

It's actually better if you quit drinking sodas at all since it's only loaded with sugar and calories. You don't gain anything beneficial for drinking it. Also, do note that fruit drinks do have a high concentration of calories, especially when it's pre-made in the stores.

If you want a fruit drink then it's best to do it on your own with natural ingredients. This way, you know what went inside of it and you know how much sugar you might be adding into your drink.

Fibrous Carbs

You want to rid yourself of any starchy carbs since it is bad for your body. If you aren't sure of what starchy carbs are, its carbs that mainly comes from junk food, which means that it's high in calories despite the small portion size.

However, other carbs like fibrous carbs can be eaten in a higher amount without the need to worry about the high amount of calories it has. Not only does it have a high water content but it also have vitamins and minerals included.

Fibrous carbs helps your digestive system run smoothly and it helps manages your blood sugar by slowing down the absorption of sugar. Basically, don't eat starchy carbs but fibrous carbs.

Winging Weight Loss

The whole point of "winging" something is to go with the flow. By not paying attention to what you eat and not planning out a daily schedule of what you are going to do for the day, you are making it harder on yourself to continue with your diet plan.

It might seem easy in the beginning because you've just started out. However, once the weeks have passed and you have not yet seen your expected results, it's time to know that you've done nothing.

All that time you spent trying to lose weight has been a waste of time because you barely lost any pounds.

If you are planning to lose weight, you cannot simply move with the flow and expect that something will happen just because you are following some instructions given to you.

Even worse, it is possible that you might even obtain excessive weight because you weren't being careful enough about your own weight. The reason why planning is so important during a diet is so you will have a clear idea of what to do.

You are not going to miss any step along the way and that you're mentally and physically prepared for the next obstacle that you will face.

If you're simply "winging" it then it's time you reconsider what you want to do and how motivated you are into losing weight. Don't waste your time if you're not going to be fully committed.

Conclusion

Now that you've reached the end of this book, there is nothing left that you need to know. If you've been keeping up with this program throughout the whole book then you should start seeing some results right about now.

You need to work hard in order to lose your weight and you need to work hard to maintain it once you've reached your goal.

In weight loss, your goal will never stop ending. You will always have a new goal in your mind, whether it is to stay active or to lose a few more pounds.

If anything, you can even put yourself back into the beginning of this book and pretend that you're a novice once more.

Remember to always stay active and to eat healthy no matter where you are or what you're doing. Keep up a schedule and a workable plan for the rest of your life.

If you start to make your health a priority in your life, you will have a much easier time going through the weight loss program once more.

Good luck and have fun.